"I'M TIRED TOO"

"I'm Tired Too"

A Guide to Chronic Fatigue Syndrome

RAEYA BOGNAR

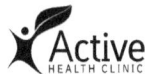

Active Health Clinic

"I'm Tired Too"

A Guide to Chronic Fatigue Syndrome

RAEYA BOGNAR

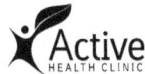

Active Health Clinic

Contents

Dedication

This book is for the previous version of me that had such a
hard time with my illness.
This book is also for you, and for every person I have ever
worked with, you've taught me everything I know, and
everything I aspire to be.
For all the unknown, you know yourself best, don't doubt
it, trust it and let it guide you.
Your journey is yours, own it, craft it
Your journey, your story.

Foreword

This book aims to be hope, light and guidance.

To the person with the diagnosis – I hope this empowers you to understand not only you and your diagnosis, but also your pathway and strategy.

To the person reading because of a loved one – I hope you are able to better understand the myriad of challenges, emotions and overall hurdles that one faces with a diagnosis such as ME/CFS or *any* invisible illness.

I will only account to what I know, personally and professionally, but the hope of this book is to share awareness, light, provide support, empathy and understanding, and hopefully have a ripple effect.

In my darkest days and hours, I made myself 2 promises: If I ever got better, that I'll make up for all the time I lost, and if I'm ever in a better position, that I would help as many people through this journey as possible.

Where it started
for me

There's a day that you wake up and you realise that the fatigue from yesterday hasn't lifted. Then you start to think about that and realise the fatigue didn't lift yesterday either. You continue to think, and realise it's been quite a while since you woke up without feeling like you had been hit by a bus, which makes you feel like you've been hit by a bus all over again. You roll over and go back to sleep, because today is already too challenging. You wake up a few hours later; starving, thirsty, needing to pee, and utterly exhausted, today is not your day. When you're finally able to start your day *roll over and doom scroll on your phone to wake up*, it doesn't fully distract you from all the symptoms you're already feeling. The day is half done, and you haven't left bed yet.

That was my experience for 270 days, before someone could tell me what was going on. Each morning, I woke up hoping that today would be the day I felt great, and it was all just a phase, but 9 months is too long to be a phase, is it not?

The blood tests revealed Epstein-Barr Virus (EBV). "No, you don't have it right now, you've had it sometime, but it's definitely the cause of your fatigue." That was 6 months ago though...? Surely it can't be that anymore?

It took 9 months, and 8 doctors, before someone uttered the phrase "It could be Chronic Fatigue Syndrome (CFS), but that's really rare and it's unlikely". This was my Mum's Women's Health Doctor, who suggested I see a Paediatrician. So off I went, excited for some answers, finally a direction, finally someone who might understand... "Yep you have Chronic Fatigue Syndrome, but I'm afraid there's not too much known about it, we'll do our best". This lead to another referral, which lead to a hospital in-patient rehabilitation program where I was told I would get better, "You are young, you will be fine", which gave me false hope, and not answers, or information, it gave me strategies, but not how to adapt and mould them to my needs.

5 years... from the age of 14 to 19, that's 1,825 days that I was missing from my life. At that stage 25% of my entire life had been spent with overwhelming, life-impacting fatigue.

I couldn't go to school, I couldn't work, I couldn't socialise, I couldn't play sport, I couldn't "be a good friend". I was fighting each day to exist and deal with an internal invisible battle within my body and my existence. It's important for me to note that my journey is generally discussed as age 14-19. It didn't stop there, but at the age of 19, life became more accessible. I had a change in circumstances, some more help, some more information, guidance and wisdom, which meant my journey changed course.
In hindsight, I feel that from the age of 19-23 I really gaslit myself into believing that I was better than I was, but life was so damn amazing now that I could walk, work, socialise and help. It charged me, it became the new me. I was still booming and busting, but it was for a cause, it was worth it.

I am one of the individuals that did get better, but instead of saying "recovered" or "cured" (ewwww), I now say, "I currently no longer fit the diagnostic criteria for CFS". Because it's true, I don't, but saying things this way highlights that I still need to live my life in a way that is supportive of my history of CFS. I pace, I listen to my body, I do right by my health, I know where my limits are, and I know how to support them. This is what every crash, every boom, every appointment, every learning, has taught me. It has slowly built and accumulated to the version of me that I am today and the toolkit that I have.

In this book, we're not going to talk about me. It's not about me. This is my view, experience, and expertise in understanding and managing CFS - the overview of considerations, if you will. This is not health advice, but rather an expression of experience and understanding. Take what applies to you and seek clarifications on the rest from other supports. My hope is that this book gives insight and brings visibility to something otherwise invisible.

Chapter 1

Known Knowns, Known Unknowns, and Unknown Unknowns...

There could not be a more accurate statement to CFS, there are things we know about it, things we know that we do not know about it, and there is still so much unknown that we don't know what we don't know yet.

How's your brain fog? Have I lost you?

Why is this important? It's the reason, probably one of many, as to why each person's journey is so very different, and why it is not, and cannot be, a one-size-fits-all approach to understanding, connecting dots or management of the condition. This is also your first reminder that no one person, thing, program or product can solely cater to your needs. There are Biopsychosocial elements to your needs, and therefore you need a multidisciplinary team to help you manage your way through.

Let's start with the unknown unknowns...

This one is short and sweet - we simply haven't figured these things out yet...
This doesn't mean you're stuck, but it does mean that research and evidence is still evolving. This means it will still be labelled as a neurological "syndrome" because not all the answers are there yet. We also have good evidence to suggest that there are most likely different types of Myalgic Encephalomyelitis/ Chronic Fatigue Syndrome (ME/CFS) - in terms of the physiological process and understanding. This is in addition to understanding what we know about the nervous system and its role in all of this too. We don't know the cause, but we know the effect (impact).
And put simply - we don't know what we don't know - yet...

Now the known unknowns... maybe that was accidentally already covered?

There's a lot that we know we don't know, such as some of the biomechanics and physiological evidence behind what's happening within ME/CFS. This is heavily debated in the academic world, even ME versus CFS, which some believe is one and the same, and others believe are two completely different conditions. The answer to this? It depends where you are and who you are talking to. Some countries use the terms interchangeably, as do some people, and others believe they are separate conditions, with differing severities. I am not here to weigh in on this debate, either way, they both fall under chronic invisible illnesses which need more validation, understanding, support, empathy, and funding!!

The cause may be unknown for now, but the effect has been heavily discussed. Again, not the whole answer, but there is evidence to suggest that ME/CFS leads to an increased allostatic load on the body (which is a fancy term for physiological stress), which can then lead to a dysregulated nervous system and as a result, central sensitisation, all of which can lead to other co-morbidities and associated symptoms.

What do we know?
We have several factors that predispose us to a chronic invisible illness. These can be, but are not limited to:

- Genetics & Epigenetics
- Autonomic or BP dysregulation syndromes
- Hypermobility disorders
- Adverse childhood events
- History of trauma
- Personality types or traits
- Lifestyle factors
- Mental health conditions
- Thyroid and/or Iron conditions
- Mast Cell Disorders such as Mast Cell Activation Syndrome (MCAS)
- Disordered eating, food intolerances
- Neurodivergence
- Central Sleep Disorders

· Other chronic health issues

Having these doesn't automatically result in getting ME/CFS: you may have one or many, but generally, we have these things which predispose us to a chronic illness. Then we tend to have factors that challenge our health, our nervous system, bring on symptoms and exacerbate what may be lurking under the surface. We call these precipitating factors or our triggers.

Triggers can be anything, again, commonly we'll see;

· Infections
· Illnesses
· Physical/Emotional stress and/or trauma
· Injuries
· Concussions
· Significant life events: changes, disruptions
· Unmanaged / Unknown health conditions

These can be singular, multiple (at once or over time), acute or chronic and ongoing.

What are the other factors you ask? Well, co-morbidities are also another interesting discussion, and to be honest, almost anything can be a co-morbidity to ME/CFS, because any health challenge can predispose us to experiencing ME/CFS and can also exacerbate ME/CFS symptoms.

The common comorbidities we see alongside ME/CFS are:

- Chronic Pain Syndromes
- Autonomic Nervous System Dysfunction (Dysautonomia)
- Sleep Disorders
- Long-COVID - Post-Acute Sequalae of Covid (PASC)
- Hypermobility Spectrum Disorders
- Neurodivergence
- Autoimmune conditions
- Mental health conditions: Anxiety, Depression, Trauma, PTSD, and pretty much all of them
- My AHC Dietitian family will kill me if I don't include gastrointestinal issues/conditions, allergies, intolerances, MCAS etc.
- And many, many more

Why are the known knowns important? Well, it's important to know that you're not the "unlucky" one to fall ill. It's not random or chance, it's a series of factors and circumstances that come together to have the impact that they do.

Lastly in the known, knowns... symptoms.
Did you know that there are around 100 symptoms that are considered "common" in ME/CFS, and even MORE in Long-COVID. It doesn't mean that they're "normal", but my point is, ME/CFS is not just fatigue.

"Common" symptoms include:

- Debilitating Fatigue: mental and/ or physical
- Cognitive Dysfunction: brain fog - thinking, concentration and memory challenges
- Post-Exertion Malaise - challenges recovering from exertion
- Unrefreshing sleep / Sleep challenges

^ These are the diagnostic criteria for ME/CFS, in addition to experiencing one or more of:

- Myalgia (muscle pain)
- Arthralgia (joint pain)
- Sore throats
- Tender glands
- Flu-like symptoms
- Headaches & Migraines
- Sensitivity to noise
- Sensitivity to light
- Sensitivity to standing
- Sensitivity to temperature
- Altered appetite
- And many, many more

To understand symptoms, we also must understand how much they fluctuate. An ME/CFS patient will experience 'baseline' symptoms daily. This is what they learn to function around.

Even if you see them up and about, it doesn't mean they're symptom free, it means the symptoms are at a level they can manage. Symptoms will fluctuate, so on a bad day or in a flare up/crash, symptoms will get worse and more of them will come. On a standard day, the average ME/CFS patient is likely to experience 4-6 symptoms, and on a bad day they can have as many as 10-20, these can fluctuate and vary or could be all at once. Symptoms are invisible, which is why an ME/CFS patient will always get told "but you look fine". This isn't reassuring, nor is it a compliment, it's actually *very* invalidating.

Let's talk about me as an example: Every. Single. Day. I woke up from a very bad sleep, already exhausted, my body ached, my head hurt and was slow, my legs were sore, and I was dizzy. That's an average day, that's 7 symptoms, that was every day, that's 1,825 days (conservatively), that's minimum 12 hours a day, that's almost 22,000 hours of symptoms. The person who said that your teens years are the prime of your life, clearly didn't have my experience.

Now, let's talk about a bad day. I'd wake up after anywhere from 12-16 hours of (bad) sleep: tired, exhausted, with a headache, sore throat, achy body, brain fog, no appetite, weak, dizzy, light-headed, fast heart rate, and sensitivity to light & noise; I would struggle with standing, my joints were in pain, and I felt like I had the flu. That's double the number of symptoms from an average day. Do you know how often this happened? Weekly. Anywhere from 1 day a week to the entire week itself. My symptoms fluctuated, therefore my capacity did too. It meant that each day I had no idea what I was capable of, how long the symptoms were going to last and what I could do about it. It was like the worst version of Groundhog Day.

My case is just one example, and these conditions impact everyone differently. My main point is; symptoms vary in severity, intensity, frequency, significance, type, duration and recovery. Meaning that the "tools" that help them will vary just as much.
This is a reminder that you cannot judge a diagnosis, nor should you! It is important to understand how the illness impacts the person, and how the person impacts the illness.

This book aims to support you in your journey, whether that be your own diagnosis, or supporting a loved one through theirs.

Chapter 2

Step One - Your Roadmap

Now that we're a little clearer on what's going on here, let's get to what this book is meant to be about – how to practically support yourself on this journey.

Firstly, you need to know your story, you need to understand, to rule in and rule out all other health conditions.

ME/CFS is only diagnosed once the person has been experiencing symptoms for 6+ months, or 3+ months in the case of adolescence and children. It is also a diagnosis of exclusion, so you will get tests, do assessments and be asked questions, once the medical provider is confident nothing else is going on, you will be diagnosed.

With or without diagnosis, you will need a team around you. This may include those within your home and family/friend/ peer supports, as well as a medical team. A GP should and can act as your case manager, help you with symptom management, investigate and diagnose comorbidities, and provide referrals to the appropriate people. Your team will be dependent on your symptoms; Light-headed? Dizzy? High heart rate? You'll need to see a Cardiologist. Injuries? Pain? You'll need to see someone to check on hypermobility. Ongoing joint and muscle pain? A Rheumatologist. This list will go on and on.

Having a roadmap to help you navigate your care is one of the key components to understanding not only your illness, but also your pathway, your journey. Understanding your health conditions and challenges will help you to receive diagnosis, treatment, validation and assist you to find your foundations, your pillars and your people.

Below is a list of provider types and the help they may be able to supply.

Medical

- Cardiology/Electrophysiology - Heart conditions and dysautonomia diagnosis and management.
- Clinical Psychology - Mental health support.
- Endocrinology - Diagnosis and treatment/management of conditions that impact endocrine system and hormones.
- Gastroenterology - Diagnosis and treatment/management of conditions affecting digestive system.
- Geneticist - Diagnosis and management of genetic and hereditary conditions.

- Gynaecology - Diagnosis and treatment/management of conditions of the reproductive system of those assigned female at birth (AFAB).
- Immunology/Allergy - Diagnosis and treatment/ management of immune problems such as food allergies, seasonal allergies and immunodeficiencies
- Neurology - Diagnosis and treatment/management of conditions of the brain, spinal cord and nerves.
- Nurse Practitioner - a Registered Nurse with a special, post-graduate qualification that allows them to be a specialist in a particular area, run a ward on a hospital, and in some cases, prescribe medication.
- Practice Nurse - someone who works at your GP practice who will do health checks and sometimes write the (currently called) Chronic Disease Management Plan (CDM)
- Paediatrics - A doctor specializing in the health of infants, children and adolescents.
- Pharmacology - Support in dispensing and reviewing of medications and interactions etc., can conduct something called an 'independent medication review'
- General Physician/Consultant – A doctor with a wealth of experience that has not chosen to specialise formally, however, they may be a specialist in an area such as Chronic Pain, or Chronic Fatigue.
- Psychiatry - Mental health diagnosis and avenue to more advanced treatment options such as medication intervention and inpatient stays.
- Rheumatology - Diagnosis and treatment/management of conditions/diseases that impact joint/muscles/bones of both inflammatory and autoimmune nature.

Allied Health

- Allied Health Assistant
- Chiropractic
- Chinese Medicine
- Counselling
- Dietetics
- Exercise Physiology
- Myotherapy
- Naturopathy
- Occupational Therapy
- Osteopathy
- Physiotherapy
- Podiatry
- Psychology
- Social Work
- and many more, especially if you're not from Australia.

Chapter 3

Step 1.5 - The Foundations

Pacing and post-exertional malaise (PEM), Planning and Prioritising

Let's start with PEM, this can also be labelled as post-exertional neuroimmune exertion (PENE) and post-exertion symptom exacerbation (PESE). PEM is a distinctive exacerbation of symptoms and a further reduction in functioning after physical, cognitive, orthostatic (upright posture), emotional or sensory stress. In the absence of a "primary treatment" for ME/CFS, the mainstay of treatment commonly agreed upon globally, is the prevention of illness exacerbation and symptom escalation by "pacing" to prevent PEM. The better we prevent PEM, the more stable we are. Stability can be better managed, and for some, this can be the stable footing to be able to build an increased capacity from. The opposite is also true, the more we push, the more we boom and crash. PEM results in severe crashes, and overall, a decline in function. In some, this decline has been seen to be permanent.

This brings us to the concept of pacing. Understanding pacing means that we understand the different types of physiological stressors that can lead to energy expenditure. This can be physical activity, orthostatic stress, cognitive work, emotional exchanges, infection, poor sleep, and sensory input, among others. We also need to consider that the type, intensity, frequency, and duration of triggers are also considerable factors when pacing.

Unfortunately, I can only be nice and general in this book, but I can remind you that managing this is an exceptionally challenging process. If it was possible for you to read a book and be better by it, the book would already exist, and the person who wrote it would be making millions. As I said earlier, there is no one size fits all approach to this concept, so meet with knowledgeable health professionals, curate a team, ask for help, and learn your way through this.

Back to pacing, it is as unique as your beautiful self is. I like to call this the goldilocks theory; there is too much, there is too little, and then there is your baseline which is something in between. Your diagnosis and conditions, and the symptoms you struggle with the most, will influence what you feel you can and cannot do. Likewise, if you have 10 different diagnoses, or are neurodivergent, or a solo parent, or 2 years or 20 years into your journey, this will influence how you pace, how you engage in activity and how you rest. I always suggest that you explore this in a deeper way, to better understand finding your version of pacing. Leaning in to understanding pacing, and better understanding yourself, can only lead to better symptom management, and, ideally, stability - and then maybe even progression.

My first bit of general advice? Build your pacing concepts around your bad days - around the 'current' or realistic version of yourself, not your good days, your goals, or your idealistic version of yourself. The nature of these conditions is that they vary day to day. Try to take control of the factors you can control, which will help you to gently influence the factors that you cannot control. Take it from me, the self-proclaimed "Queen of what not to do", to the now self-proclaimed "Queen of pacing". Someone get me a throne. To this day, I am adamant that my booming and busting, my pushing my body, my expectations of my body, of my health, is the reason I got as disabled and debilitated as I did. It wasn't until I learnt the art of pacing that I was able to get some control back, that I was able to settle the storm of symptoms, and that I was able to create change. This comes back to the earlier statement - avoid and prevent PEM, focus on pacing.

Pacing is intimate, it is yours. It's okay if you've tried something and it hasn't worked for you, it's all about furthering your understanding. Learn what it is you don't know and get support for what it is you struggle with. Understand your personal triggers; there will be themes, but also uniqueness to them as yours. All information is helpful, learning the hard way (like me) is sucky, but in the end, it's further data to help you move forwards. You don't know what you don't know yet, remember?

This brings me to planning and prioritising. Pacing is planning, it's prioritising, it is the balance of the hierarchy of needs. Understanding your baseline (what you can do in one day and repeat the next day without PEM) helps you to understand your capacity, as well as your triggers. This also will help you to organise what you have to, want to, or need to prioritise, and it can also mean that you can have planning and structure to your days, and work towards consistency. Again, not a one-size-fits-all approach. This is general advice from both my personal and professional experience, but as is the age old saying, this is where the gold is.

As my doctor indicated, we didn't have a great pathway, there wasn't a whole lot of understanding or help (at that point in time), which meant that I didn't really feel validated, understood, or even seen. The many passing comments I received like; "aren't you better yet?", "but you don't look sick", "have you tried *this*, surely *this* will fix you". I felt broken, I felt inadequate, and I felt alone, so alone. Since working as a practitioner, I've really noticed how fundamental validation, understanding and empathy are in this journey, as well as how challenging things like independence are, or managing the isolation, or the regular identity crisis. Have you ever had a day where you have a really exciting plan, and then you wake up sick and can't go? The disappointment, the betrayal and the realisation of how little control we have in that moment? That's every day in the life of ME/CFS. It strips your identity, it strips your independence, and it isolates you from not only who you thought you were, but who you want to be and what and who you want to be around.

Coming back to the chapter title, the foundations. The foundations are not only pacing. The foundations are also community, understanding and empathy, so that you have a shining light in what is a very dark tunnel, guiding the way, or holding your hand when there's a stumble.

Chapter 4

Step Two - The Pillars

Health is wealth, and we don't realise how important this is to us, until it's taken away and we miss something we no longer have, well at least, that was my experience. This book is about reminding you how important your health is, how important you are. This journey is a challenging one. This book is to help you understand the pathways, and help you navigate the terrain. Again, with my very general advice, the pillars to me are; understanding your symptom profile, your diagnosis, your triggers, your recharge strategies, your capacity, your team and their roles.

I don't have all the answers for you, but I do believe that the first step of understanding your diagnosis and your symptom profile, will help with validation, and taking your health seriously. This will help you work towards health ownership - whatever that may look like to you.

Understanding your triggers and recharge strategies will help you better understand your capacity. This helps you to acknowledge realistic standards and expectations on your current body and health circumstances to then build out from there.

Your triggers; these are what exacerbate your symptoms or cause you PEM. These can be physical and orthostatic, cognitive and emotional, social, environmental and sensory stress. Triggers vary from person to person and can (and will) change throughout your journey, so knowing them is extremely important. Also important to note is that some things can be a trigger sometimes, and not other times; the complexity is in the context. Triggers can also be; things that you see, hear, smell, taste, touch, people, places, things you say/think/believe, and things happening in your body. Triggers can be subtle and only noticeable to the person experiencing them and result in a slight change in their symptoms, or they can be exceptionally obvious and lead to significant booming and busting.

Contrary to triggers, we have restorative practices and activities. Theoretically, these are what we need to use, to offset and support exposure to triggers. We know that we can't and shouldn't hide ourselves away from all triggers, but we also know we can't dive headfirst into them either. Like triggers, we have physical, cognitive, emotional, social and sensory forms of rest. In addition, "energy" or "capacity" is transient - it's not a black and white concept, there's grey and everything in between. I explain this as negative, neutral and positive energy expenditure. We have activities that take energy, we have things that will give energy, and we'll have things that will do both, which will sit in more of a neutral category. Work/Study/ Cleaning = energy negative, Resting/Mindfulness/TV Shows = energy positive, Craft/Socialising/Hobbies = energy neutral - they will give and take. Understanding where activities fit for you helps you to better understand your overall baseline principles.

Understanding your baseline, I have already touched on, but this is where I have the least amount of advice to give to *you* specifically. You can Google and understand triggers or restorative practices, but you can't Google what your personal baseline is. This took me quite some time to figure out, and it also took me time to understand how, and why, to respect it. Health professionals, Google and peers will be able to give you a rough idea of what your baseline may be, but it will require some exploration on your part too. One thing I will try to remind you of; when you find it, whatever it may be, please show yourself, and your body, compassion. Nobody, I repeat, *nobody*, wants to be unwell and have this condition, so be your own cheerleader and your support person, not your harshest critic.

And lastly, have your team, and know their role. There are these age-old sayings "Rome wasn't built in a day" or "it takes a village to raise a child". This is also true for your health journey. You won't miraculously recover in a day, and you also won't be able to do this alone, nor should you expect yourself to go through something so challenging and life altering on your own. As mentioned in Chapter 2, you will need a team for guidance, support, diagnosis & treatment. In addition to a team, having community and collaboration will go a long way in supporting you in this journey.

It would be amiss of me if I didn't acknowledge that there are 3 themes when it comes to navigating complex and challenging health circumstances; isolation, identity and independence - regardless of the person's background. In my career, I've had the privilege of working with many, many people. To date I've had over 5,000 hours of clinical experience, and over 50,000 hours of personal experience. I've worked with people from the age of 6, to over the age of 90, I've worked with people face-to-face, and internationally, even those where English is their second language. I've worked with people with a clean record when it comes to their health, and people with decades of trauma, and everything in between. With all this personal and professional experience and working at an incredible clinic that strives to not only make invisible illnesses, visible, but prides itself on integrity, access, community and more, a common theme we see that is exceptionally important in this journey, is validation.

3 key themes:

Isolation:
I mentioned earlier that I went "missing" from my life. What I mean by this was yes, I still existed, but the version of me that I was, that I wanted to be, was no longer accessible. I was missing from sport, school, socialising and I simply couldn't live as the version of me that I truly was and wanted to be and do what I wanted to do. I was incredibly isolated. Not only could I no longer do those things, but I also no longer felt like myself. I didn't feel understood, I didn't feel seen, I wasn't connected or engaged, and I didn't have a community behind me. Remember my reference to "Rome" and a "Village"? I didn't have these things, and it was incredibly isolating to experience.

Identity:
I've definitely touched on this point already, but have you ever gone through a period of life where you no longer feel like you? That you don't want to, or can't do the things you usually do? Has it made you question your decisions? Your understanding of things or life? Your understanding of you? This is what it's like in ME/CFS. You have this previous version of you that is no longer accessible, you have parts of life that are no longer accessible, but you have this framework of what you have been, things that you have done and that has just vanished. Your blueprint no longer matches up, and it's like you must learn anew, in a new world, with none of the superpowers you used to have. Not only is this incredibly disconcerting, we have no framework or understanding of how to manage this, and we also generally don't feel we have a pathway throughout it all. Like I mentioned earlier, you wake up every day, hoping,

wishing, maybe even praying - both to a God you may believe in, or hoping that even if you don't, you're desperate enough to try it anyway.

You have a previous version of yourself, you have this current, unidentifiable version of yourself and then you have this hopeful and idealistic version of you that you want to be, and maybe desperately try to be. You're trying to make space for all 3 of them in your brain and on any given day have the identity crisis behind which one is being true to you and who you are. It's isolating, it's challenging, and none of this comes in a handy textbook to tell us how to get through it.

Independence:
The above brings me to one of the final pieces, of the challenges, unfortunately not the overall puzzle. Isolation and lack of clarity behind identity may mean you desperately crave independence. You desperately crave understanding and the ability to take control. Alas, independence is another illusive part of this illness. ME/CFS strips away your capacity, your tolerance of previous likes/loves/challenges has altered, you now have triggers, you now have PEM, and you have a very delicate balance of managing the two. ME/CFS is the delicate balance of wanting, needing, and having to do things, and how to balance the triggers and recovery on the other side. This alters what we can do, and what we have access to, which then significantly impacts our independence, and who we are. When our body feels like it is independently controlling all elements of our life, we struggle to manage not only daily activities but also meaningful activities.

Then, there's the grief, of who you were, who you wanted to be, who you think you can be, the things we could do, the people that were there, and all the rest. This is not to scare you, nor to paint a solely negative light on it all, rather to discuss how complex and complicated this journey is. And maybe to the person reading, if you're going through this journey, I hope that you feel seen and heard, validated and understood. To the person who hasn't, maybe you get this a little better than you have before.

It's not just tired, it's not even just the fatigue, it's everything else...

Chapter 5

The Upgrades & Beyond

You may be 5,000 words deep and questioning the point of this book - I wouldn't blame you.

To summarise, the key message here is to better understand not only you and your diagnosis, and your pathway and strategy, but maybe also for someone who doesn't have these conditions, to better understand the myriad of challenges, emotions and overall hurdles that one faces with a diagnosis such as ME/CFS or *any* invisible illness. I can only account to what I know, personally and professionally, but the hope of this book is to share awareness, light, provide support, empathy and understanding, and hopefully have a ripple effect. In my darkest days and hours, I made myself 2 promises: If I ever got better, that I'll make up for all the time I lost, and if I'm ever in a better position, that I would help as many people through this journey as possible. I also very wholeheartedly believe in being the change we wish to see in the world, so I put my thoughts on paper, in the hopes that it helps one person, and that they also may help one person, and together, invisible becomes more visible. In my lifetime, I hope that I see this space, the invisible illness space, to be more understood, validated, and supported.

What worked for me may not work for you, or the next person, but I urge you to not focus on fitting the mould, rather on building and planting your pathway, writing your story, and being open to learning, evolving and owning your journey. The upgrades to the pillars and beyond are easily summarised like this: always strive on learning, growing and building. That progression isn't just in the quantity and quality of what it is you can do or how you may feel, but also the tools you have in the tool kit, the PEM you've prevented, the wins you've achieved, the chapters and chapters of knowledge you've learnt through experience, and the amazing person you were, are, and will continue to be regardless of diagnosis, capacity or story. May I remind you, regardless of setbacks, flare ups, relapses, you can never be back to a starting point or square one. Each day you know more, each month you're managing your tools in your tool kit, each year, you're mastering your knowledge and skills. please don't discredit this because you're "still sick", or "still have symptoms". You are incredible, and amazing, and all of the positive compliments, not because I'm toxically positive, but because you are you, and this is difficult, and you STILL show up.

You are not alone, you are not an exception, you don't have to be misunderstood or invalidated, there are people, places, services, books, podcasts, webinars that exist to help you understand you and your journey. It may take some time to find your team, your village and your tools but they are out there.

The power is yours, not in being able to influence or control your diagnosis, rather the ownership of your journey, it is yours, you are you. In the wise words of Winnie the Pooh "You are braver than you believe, stronger than you seem and smarter than you think". The other, wise words I have for you; "Everything will be ok in the end, if it's not okay, it's not the end".

Lastly, for the person reading who chose to read this to better understand a loved one's diagnosis, thank-you. Secondly, be the person your loved one *needs* you to be, not who you think you should be, you're not living in their body, let *them* guide *you*. When in doubt, when you have questions, when you don't understand, ask, don't assume. Be their support, be their cheer-leader, and be the change you want to see in the world.

Dr Seuss once said "No one is you, that is truer than true, there is no one alive who is youer than you". You have the choice to be you and who that is. Choose to be a support, an ally, an advocate, and to help someone be them too. Choose love, support, empathy, validation and understanding. I also want to acknowledge that this can, and will be hard on you too, especially if your person, your loved one is suffering in this journey. I hope you better understand their journey, and I encourage you, to seek your own support, to have your own team, we're humans, not made of steel, you will need help, and that's okay.

You've got this.

Learn more...

Head to our social media channel (Instagram, Facebook, YouTube and Tik Tok) to learn more tips and tricks to manage your fatigue.

Watch this Youtube video to learn more about Raeya's journey with ME/CFS through the years.

Have you done our "Missing diagnosis quiz?" It's a short quiz that helps a person identify their symptom profile and categorise where their symptoms fit within their diagnosis and what they may need around that.